CONGNITIVE BEHAVIOURA L THERAPY

A Comprehensive Guide To Cognitive Behavioral Therapy For Lasting Mental Wellness And Personal Growth

WILFREDO CARSON

INTRODUCTION

Cognitive Behavioral Therapy (CBT) is a well-known and commonly used style of psychotherapy that is beneficial in the treatment of a variety of mental health conditions. This therapeutic method is based on the notion that thoughts, feelings, and behaviors are interrelated and that by changing maladaptive thought patterns, people can improve their emotional well-being. This detailed examination will delve into the core components of CBT, beginning with an overview and progressing to a historical viewpoint to trace its growth. The theoretical foundations of CBT will then be examined to better comprehend the psychological concepts that underpin this treatment method.

1.1 An Overview of Cognitive Behavioral Therapy:

Cognitive Behavioral Therapy is a therapeutic method that employs both cognitive and behavioral techniques to address and improve dysfunctional thought patterns and behaviors. The core concept of cognitive behavioral therapy is that people's perceptions of situations have a major impact on their emotional responses and subsequent behaviors. CBT strives to uncover and confront harmful thought patterns through therapist-client collaboration, replacing them with healthier, more adaptive beliefs.

The behavioral component of CBT is developing ways to change negative behaviors, reinforcing positive acts, and supporting the development of coping mechanisms. This comprehensive approach identifies CBT as a goal-oriented, problem-solving therapy with strong scientific backing across a wide range of mental health conditions.

1.2 Historical Development of CBT:

Cognitive Behavioral Therapy originated in the mid-twentieth century as a response to the limitations of traditional psychoanalytic and behavioral treatments. Psychologists such as Albert Ellis and Aaron T. Beck established the groundwork for CBT by questioning the dominant beliefs about the significance of unconscious processes. In the 1950s, Albert Ellis created Rational Emotive Behavior Therapy (REBT), which emphasized the importance of irrational beliefs in psychological suffering.

In the 1960s, Beck introduced Cognitive Therapy, which focused on cognitive restructuring to treat depression symptoms. These pioneering works laid the groundwork for the combination of cognitive and behavioral concepts, which resulted in the establishment of Cognitive Behavioral Therapy as a unique therapeutic modality. CBT has evolved over the years, including aspects from numerous psychological theories, and is now a widely utilized and empirically validated technique for treating a wide range of mental health conditions.

1.3 Theoretical Basis of CBT:

Cognitive Behavioral Therapy's theoretical foundations are based on a variety of psychological theories, combining cognitive and behavioral concepts to address the interaction of thoughts, emotions, and behaviors. Cognitive theory holds that erroneous and maladaptive cognitive patterns contribute to emotional suffering. Beck's Cognitive Therapy, for example, established the concept of cognitive distortions, which include patterns like catastrophizing, black-and-white thinking, and overgeneralization. This cognitive component is supported by the behavioral approach, which emphasizes the importance of learned behaviors in generating psychological well-being. The incorporation of these theories within CBT provides for a more complete understanding of the reciprocal relationship between cognitive processes and behavior, providing a sophisticated foundation for therapeutic intervention.

The emphasis on empirical validation, as well as the incorporation of aspects from learning theories like operant and classical conditioning, strengthens CBT's theoretical basis.

In conclusion, Cognitive Behavioral Therapy is a dynamic and successful therapeutic technique with a long history and solid theoretical foundations. Its history from Ellis and Beck's ground-breaking work to its current prominence as a mainstream psychotherapy modality demonstrates its versatility and reactivity to the changing landscape of mental health treatment. As we go more into the subtle components of CBT, it becomes clear that its success stems from the integration of cognitive and behavioral principles, which provides a comprehensive and evidence-based framework for addressing a wide range of mental health issues.

CHAPTER 1
UNDERSTANDING COGNITIVE BEHAVIOURAL THERAPY

Definition and Core Concepts

Cognitive Behavioral Therapy (CBT) is a commonly used therapy approach based on the idea that an individual's ideas, feelings, and behaviors are all interconnected. It works under the assumption that changing maladaptive thought patterns and behaviors can improve emotional well-being. In the context of CBT, cognition refers to the mental processes involved in learning and comprehending information. This encompasses perception, attention, memory, and problem-solving. In contrast, behavior refers to an individual's observable activities and reactions to diverse stimuli.

The Cognitive Model

The cognitive model is a core component of CBT, stressing the importance of cognition in determining emotions and behaviors. Automatic thoughts, a critical component of this approach, are spontaneous and immediate cognitions that arise in reaction to certain conditions. These thoughts frequently influence emotions and behaviors, demonstrating the interconnectedness of cognitive processes. Core beliefs, another component of the cognitive model, are strongly held and essential views about oneself, others, and the universe. These beliefs influence one's worldview and can be adaptive or maladaptive. Intermediate beliefs serve as a bridge between instinctive thoughts and core beliefs, representing conditional assumptions and behavioral guidelines.

The Behavioral Model

In addition to the cognitive model, CBT contains the behavioral model, which acknowledges the influence of external variables on an individual's psychological well-being. Classical conditioning, a notion linked with behavioral treatment, is the connection of stimuli with specific responses. This associative learning mechanism aids in the formation of emotional responses.

Operant conditioning emphasizes the consequences of behavior, reinforcing or punishing behaviors based on their outcomes. The third component of the behavioral model is modeling, which is the process of learning by seeing and imitating the behaviors of others.

These behavioral principles help us understand how external factors contribute to the development and maintenance of maladaptive habits.

<u>Cognition</u>

Cognition, as defined in the context of CBT, refers to the mental processes involved in obtaining and interpreting knowledge.

This broad area encompasses a variety of cognitive functions, including perception, attention, memory, and problem-solving. Understanding cognition is critical in CBT because it serves as the foundation for detecting and changing dysfunctional thought processes. The therapy procedure includes assisting patients in recognizing distorted or unreasonable beliefs and replacing them with more realistic and adaptive ones. By treating cognition, CBT seeks to modify how people perceive and understand their events, ultimately impacting their emotional responses and behaviors.

<u>Behavior</u>

Within the context of cognitive behavioral therapy, behavior refers to an individual's visible activities and reactions to internal and external stimuli. Behavioral patterns are viewed as learned responses to certain events, and CBT attempts to improve maladaptive habits using a variety of strategies.

Therapists use a behavior-focused approach to help clients identify problematic actions and build change strategies. This part of CBT emphasizes that modifying behavior can cause adjustments in thoughts and feelings.

It highlights the interaction of internal cognitive processes and exterior behaviors, reinforcing the notion that changing one component might affect the others.

Automatic Thoughts

Automatic ideas are spontaneous and immediate cognitive processes that arise in response to certain stimuli. These ideas are frequently fleeting and unseen by humans, yet they play an important role in influencing emotions and behaviors. CBT holds that automatic thoughts are impacted by underlying fundamental beliefs and can lead to the persistence of psychological suffering. Individuals learn to identify and question automatic thoughts during therapy, replacing negative or distorted thinking patterns with more balanced and realistic alternatives. This cognitive restructuring helps to interrupt the cycle of maladaptive thinking that leads to unpleasant emotions and behaviors.

<u>Core beliefs</u>

Core beliefs are strongly held ideas about oneself, others, and the world. These beliefs emerge gradually and are frequently the result of early life experiences, influencing an individual's worldview. Core beliefs are regarded as important contributors to emotional well-being in CBT because they influence how events are interpreted and automatic thoughts are generated. Maladaptive core beliefs, such as poor self-perceptions or gloomy views of the world, can exacerbate mental health problems.

Individuals use therapeutic therapies to investigate and confront their underlying ideas, creating more adaptive and constructive ways of thinking.

<u>Intermediate beliefs.</u>

In the CBT cognitive paradigm, intermediate beliefs serve as a bridge between automatic thoughts and core beliefs. These beliefs are the conditional assumptions and norms that govern conduct in specific contexts. Intermediate beliefs shape reactions to individual circumstances, whereas fundamental beliefs are broader and overarching. They serve as filters for instinctive thinking and contribute to the overall cognitive processing of events.

By addressing intermediate beliefs, CBT tries to reveal the conditional nature of particular thought patterns and assist individuals in developing more flexible and adaptable responses to changing conditions.

Classical Conditioning

Classical conditioning, a notion connected with the behavioral model of CBT, is the connection of stimuli with specific reactions. This type of learning, developed by Ivan Pavlov, shows how environmental signals can become associated with emotional or behavioral responses. In the therapeutic setting, classical conditioning explains how specific stimuli might elicit automatic thinking and emotional responses. CBT therapies, such as exposure therapy, aim to change these learned connections, desensitizing people to previously anxiety-provoking stimuli. By severing the link between specific stimuli and unpleasant reactions, CBT tries to reduce distress and encourage more adaptive responses.

<u>Operant Conditioning</u>

Another essential component in CBT's behavioral model is operant conditioning, which focuses on the consequences of behavior. Introduced by B.F. Skinner's operant conditioning investigates how behaviors are reinforced or diminished depending on the positive or negative results they cause.

CBT uses operant conditioning principles to change maladaptive behaviors by reinforcing positive acts and inhibiting negative ones. Individuals can learn to engage in activities that result in positive reinforcement using approaches such as behavioral activation, which contributes to enhanced mood and overall well-being.

Operant conditioning tactics enable people to create beneficial behavioral adjustments, thereby influencing their emotional experiences.

<u>Modeling</u>

Modeling, also known as observational learning, is the process of learning by seeing and mimicking others' actions. This notion, which is integrated into the CBT behavioral model, acknowledges the importance of social factors on behavior. Albert Bandura's social learning theory emphasizes the importance of modeling in the development and maintenance of behaviors. In the therapeutic setting, modeling is utilized to illustrate adaptive coping mechanisms and problem-solving abilities. Therapists may demonstrate effective ways of responding to pressures or difficult situations, giving clients examples to follow. Individuals develop new abilities and perspectives by introducing modeling into CBT, broadening their behavioral repertoire, and promoting positive changes in their actions and responses.

Cognitive Behavioral Therapy (CBT) is a rich tapestry of interwoven principles that address the complex relationship between thoughts, feelings, and behaviors. CBT, as defined by its cognitive and behavioral models, explores the complexities of cognition, behavior, automatic thoughts, core beliefs, intermediate beliefs, classical conditioning, operant conditioning, and modeling. Each notion contributes to a more complete understanding of the therapeutic process, highlighting the importance of a nuanced and integrated approach to mental health.

As practitioners and academics continue to develop and build on these ideas, CBT remains a dynamic and successful therapy technique that helps people navigate the intricacies of their psychological well-being.

CHAPTER 2
BASIC PRINCIPLES OF CBT

<u>Collaborative Empiricism:</u>

Collaborative empiricism is a basic tenet in Cognitive Behavioral Therapy (CBT) that emphasizes the value of a collaborative and participatory connection between the therapist and the client. This principle emphasizes the idea that treatment should be a collaborative effort, with both parties working together to investigate and comprehend the client's thoughts, feelings, and behaviors. The term "empiricism" promotes an emphasis on evidence and observable data above simply subjective perceptions. In CBT, the therapist and client conduct a systematic evaluation of the client's ideas and behaviors to determine their validity and confront any mistaken views. This collaborative technique allows clients to actively participate in their therapeutic journey, instilling a sense of autonomy and self-discovery.

<u>Goal-oriented, problem-solving approach:</u>

CBT is distinguished by its goal-oriented and problem-solving approach, which prioritizes the identification and resolution of specific issues that contribute to psychological distress. Therapists and clients work together to establish clear and achievable goals, which serve as a road map for the therapeutic process. The emphasis on goal-setting helps to direct therapy toward precise, measurable objectives, which improves intervention effectiveness. This technique also helps customers improve their problem-solving abilities, which will help them deal with current and future obstacles. Clients can work deliberately toward positive change by breaking complex challenges down into manageable components, which fosters a sense of accomplishment and empowerment.

CBT has a time limit and is structured.

CBT's time-limited and structured character distinguishes it from other therapy techniques. CBT is primarily planned to be a short-term solution, lasting a set number of sessions. This structured framework serves several functions, including increasing efficiency, focusing on specific goals, and reducing reliance on long-term therapy. The time constraint motivates both the therapist and the client to work hard, address issues quickly, and sustain momentum throughout the therapeutic process.

The organized nature entails employing specific approaches and treatments customized to the individual's needs, resulting in a methodical and targeted approach to addressing recognized difficulties.

Therapeutic Alliance:

The therapeutic alliance is an important component of CBT, stressing the collaborative and supporting connection between the therapist and the client. Unlike other traditional therapy techniques, CBT emphasizes the therapeutic connection as a key facilitator of change. The alliance is based on mutual respect, empathy, and understanding, providing a safe space for clients to examine and challenge their beliefs and actions.

A positive therapeutic partnership increases client engagement, trust, and readiness to share sensitive material. It also enables therapists to adjust interventions to the client's specific needs, resulting in a personalized and effective therapy experience. The strength of the therapeutic partnership is frequently seen as a predictor of treatment success in CBT.

<u>Evidence-Based Practices in CBT:</u>

Evidence-based practice is a core principle of CBT that emphasizes the incorporation of empirical research findings into clinical decision-making. CBT is based on a wealth of scientific evidence that supports its effectiveness in treating a variety of psychological illnesses. Therapists in CBT focus on established protocols and interventions that have been shown effective through thorough research and clinical studies. This evidence-based approach strengthens the legitimacy and dependability of CBT as a therapy modality. It also guarantees that interventions are constantly adjusted and updated based on the most recent research findings, fostering a dynamic and developing practice that is in line with the best available evidence. The incorporation of evidence-based techniques into CBT not only advances the field but also demonstrates a dedication to providing clients with the most effective and verified therapeutic procedures possible.

CHAPTER 3
THE THERAPEUTIC PROCESS

Cognitive Behavioral Therapy (CBT) uses an organized and methodical approach to help people overcome psychological suffering and dysfunctional behaviors. The initial step includes assessment and formulation, which provide a complete grasp of the client's thoughts, feelings, and actions.

Cognitive conceptualization, as a subtype of evaluation, entails detecting and investigating maladaptive cognitive patterns. This process is crucial to CBT because it emphasizes the importance of cognition in shaping emotions and behaviors. Therapists get insights into their clients' subjective experiences by identifying cognitive distortions and illogical beliefs.

Another critical component of assessment is behavioral analysis, which entails methodically assessing the causes, behaviors, and consequences of maladaptive acts.

This functional analysis aids in identifying the underlying causes of troublesome behaviors, resulting in a more detailed knowledge of the client's issues.

Through collaborative inquiry, the therapist and client identify patterns, triggers, and reinforcing processes that sustain dysfunctional cycles. This comprehensive assessment serves as the foundation for interventions that target particular cognitive and behavioral components of the client's problems.

Treatment planning in CBT is a collaborative process in which the therapist and client work together to construct a therapeutic plan. Drawing on assessment findings, the treatment plan sets specific goals and strategies for addressing identified concerns.

This phase entails prioritizing areas of concentration, taking into account the client's preferences and strengths, and developing an organized approach to meeting therapeutic goals. Treatment planning is dynamic, adjusting to the client's changing needs as therapy progresses, resulting in a flexible and responsive therapeutic environment.

Setting realistic goals is an important part of the therapy process because it ensures that clients have clear and attainable benchmarks to work towards. Goals in CBT are frequently specific, measurable, attainable, relevant, and time-bound (SMART). Setting realistic expectations boosts client motivation and creates a sense of success as progress is made. Therapists work with clients to develop objectives that are consistent with their beliefs and aspirations, fostering a sense of agency and empowerment in the therapeutic interaction.

Monitoring progress is a continual and iterative procedure in CBT that aids in the evaluation of therapy efficacy. Regular assessments enable therapists and clients to monitor changes in ideas, emotions, and actions over time. This continuous feedback loop allows for modifications to the treatment plan based on observed progress or obstacles. Monitoring progress is not limited to symptom reduction, but also includes broader indices of well-being and functioning.

This complete review ensures that therapy remains tailored to the client's changing needs, maximizing the therapeutic impact of CBT.

the therapeutic process in CBT evolves through a succession of interconnected concepts, beginning with a thorough assessment and formulation of the client's cognitive and behavioral patterns.

Cognitive conceptualization and behavioral analysis lay the groundwork for comprehending the client's difficulties, allowing for focused solutions. Treatment planning entails creating goals together and developing an organized approach to addressing specific issues, with realistic goal-setting being especially important for client motivation and involvement. Monitoring progress ensures that therapy remains dynamic and responsive, according to the client's changing needs. Together, these ideas form a complete framework that directs the therapeutic journey in CBT, supporting successful and evidence-based interventions.

CHAPTER 4
TECHNIQUES AND STRATEGIES FOR CBT

<u>Cognitive restructuring:</u>

Cognitive restructuring is a core strategy in Cognitive Behavioral Therapy (CBT) that aims to detect and challenge cognitive distortions. These distortions are unreasonable and prejudiced thoughts that cause undesirable feelings and behaviors. During the therapy process, patients learn to notice and examine their automatic thoughts, which are frequently distorted and unrealistic. Therapists assist clients in addressing these beliefs by assessing the evidence that supports or contradicts them. Individuals who undergo cognitive restructuring gain new, more balanced viewpoints, resulting in a shift in their emotional and behavioral responses.

This procedure increases self-awareness, promotes realistic thinking, and assists people in breaking the loop of negative thought patterns that contribute to psychological suffering.

<u>Thought Records:</u>

The use of thought recorders is a specialized cognitive restructuring approach. Thought records are structured worksheets that help people monitor their thoughts, feelings, and related activities. Clients are asked to record distressing occurrences, recognize automatic thoughts, and categorize their feelings. Dissecting these components allows people to obtain an understanding of the relationship between thoughts and emotions.

Thought recordings also aid in the detection of cognitive distortions, as clients learn to notice patterns in their thinking. This method provides a practical and systematic approach to cognitive restructuring, allowing people to effectively question and reframe maladaptive thinking.

Behavioral activation:

Behavioral activation is a key method in CBT that focuses on boosting participation in rewarding and meaningful activities to reduce symptoms of depression and other mood disorders. This technique is based on the assumption that behavioral patterns influence emotions and that by changing habits, people can improve their moods. Therapists work with clients to find activities that provide a sense of success or joy and then create an organized strategy to incorporate these activities into everyday life. Behavioral activation breaks the cycle of withdrawal and inactivity that is commonly associated with depression, generating a sense of accomplishment and reinforcing positive emotions.

<u>Exposure Therapy:</u>

Exposure treatment is a well-known CBT strategy for treating a variety of anxiety disorders, particularly phobias and post-traumatic stress disorder (PTSD). This method entails systematically and gradually exposing individuals to frightened stimuli or events in a controlled and therapeutic setting. The goal is to desensitize people to anxiety-inducing stimuli, allowing them to face and process their concerns. Therapists work with clients to create an exposure hierarchy, beginning with less anxiety-inducing scenarios and advancing to more stressful ones. Individuals learn to accept and manage their anxiety through repeated exposure, resulting in fewer avoidance actions and less distress.

Problem-solving Skills:

CBT includes problem-solving abilities as a critical component for dealing with life's obstacles and challenges. Therapists work with clients to help them discover, define, and develop effective problem-solving strategies. This method entails breaking down larger difficulties into smaller components, assessing viable solutions, and putting an action plan in place. Problem-solving abilities in CBT enable people to tackle issues in a systematic and structured manner, generating a sense of competence and self-efficacy.

Clients who learn these skills are better prepared to deal with life's challenges and setbacks, which leads to greater mental health.

<u>Relaxation and mindfulness techniques:</u>

Relaxation and mindfulness strategies are important in CBT because they help manage stress, anxiety, and other emotional disorders. These strategies are designed to increase people's awareness of the current moment while also encouraging relaxation. Therapists offer clients a variety of techniques for managing physiological arousal and reducing stress, including deep breathing, gradual muscle relaxation, and guided visualization. Mindfulness, a practice based on meditation, promotes nonjudgmental awareness of thoughts and feelings.

By implementing these practices into their daily lives, people can enhance their emotional regulation, and focus, and build a sense of serenity in the face of life's hardships.

the approaches and strategies used in Cognitive Behavioral Therapy are various and customized to certain parts of cognitive and behavioral patterns. Cognitive restructuring and thought recorders aim to correct skewed thinking, whereas behavioral activation highlights the importance of engaging activities in for mood recovery. Exposure therapy addresses anxiety by methodical confrontation of anxieties, and problem-solving abilities provide individuals with the tools they need to face life's obstacles. Finally, relaxation and mindfulness practices help to regulate emotions and focus on the present moment. The incorporation of these strategies within the CBT framework emphasizes the comprehensive and customized nature of this therapy approach, supporting the development of effective coping mechanisms and long-term improvements in mental well-being.

CHAPTER 5
APPLICATIONS OF CBT

Cognitive Behavioral Therapy (CBT) is used to treat a wide range of mental health illnesses, demonstrating its versatility and effectiveness in addressing a variety of psychological concerns. Depression and anxiety disorders are two of the most common disorders for which CBT has shown significant benefit. CBT is a leading treatment for generalized anxiety disorder (GAD). This treatment method is distinguished by its emphasis on identifying and confronting illogical attitudes and beliefs that contribute to excessive concern. CBT effectively manages anxiety symptoms by assisting individuals via cognitive restructuring and the incorporation of behavioral methods. Furthermore, in the setting of panic disorder, cognitive behavioral therapy (CBT) is critical in reducing recurring and unexpected panic attacks. Therapists who use CBT collaborate with clients to uncover and improve maladaptive thought processes associated with panic, ultimately breaking the cycle of worry.

CBT is effective in treating social anxiety disorder, which is another type of anxiety disorder. This application combines exposure therapy, in which people gradually confront dreaded social situations, with cognitive restructuring to address inaccurate beliefs about social interactions.

This combination enables people to build more adaptable cognitive patterns and behavioral reactions, thereby mitigating the effects of social anxiety. Moving on to major depressive disorder (MDD), CBT has emerged as the gold standard in psychotherapy.

The therapeutic process includes identifying and addressing problematic thought patterns while also supporting clients in creating more positive and realistic views about themselves and the world around them.

Behavioral activation, a component of CBT for depression, focuses on boosting participation in meaningful activities to combat the lethargy and withdrawal that are frequently linked with depression.

CBT is also effective in treating obsessive-compulsive disorder (OCD). CBT for OCD often includes exposure and response prevention (ERP), a strategy that involves gradually exposing feared obsessions while avoiding compulsive rituals.

This technique seeks to disrupt the obsessive-compulsive cycle and alleviate the distress caused by intrusive thoughts. CBT gives people tools to question the erroneous ideas that drive obsessive behaviors and develop healthier coping mechanisms.

PTSD is distinguished by intrusive memories, avoidance, unfavorable changes in cognition and mood, and hyperarousal. CBT, especially trauma-focused CBT, is a recommended treatment for PTSD. This strategy entails gradually confronting and processing painful memories in a safe therapeutic setting. Cognitive restructuring enables individuals to rethink and adjust incorrect views about the traumatic event, resulting in a more adaptive perspective of the experience.

Eating disorders are another area where CBT has proven useful.

CBT is used to treat illnesses such as anorexia nervosa, bulimia nervosa, and binge-eating disorder by addressing distorted body image, disordered eating practices, and dysfunctional food and weight ideas.

Cognitive restructuring is critical in confronting the false ideas that underlying these disorders, whilst behavioral approaches assist individuals in developing healthier eating habits. Substance use disorders are a difficult challenge, and CBT has emerged as an effective approach for addressing the cognitive and behavioral elements of addiction.

CBT for drug use disorders entails recognizing and changing maladaptive thought patterns linked to substance use, establishing coping strategies, and increasing motivation for change. The treatment approach may also involve relapse prevention measures to assist people in navigating high-risk circumstances without resorting to substance abuse.

Chronic pain management is one area where CBT broadens its application beyond standard mental health issues.

CBT for chronic pain recognizes the interaction of physical sensations, thoughts, and emotions. People with chronic pain frequently experience increased anguish and incapacity as a result of inappropriate cognitive and emotional reactions to pain.

In this situation, CBT aims to change problematic thought patterns, promote adaptive coping techniques, and improve overall functioning. By addressing the psychological aspects of chronic pain, CBT becomes an essential component of a multidisciplinary approach to pain management, allowing people to live more fulfilled lives despite chronic pain.

Finally, Cognitive Behavioral Therapy has numerous applications that cover a wide range of mental health conditions.

CBT's adaptability stems from its capacity to address the interplay between thoughts, emotions, and behaviors, making it an effective therapy for a wide range of psychiatric illnesses. From anxiety and depression to OCD, PTSD, and eating disorders, cognitive behavioral therapy (CBT) teaches people how to question maladaptive thinking, adjust behaviors, and eventually improve their mental health. Furthermore, its application in drug use disorders and chronic pain management demonstrates CBT's comprehensive nature, expanding its reach beyond traditional psychiatric areas. As the area of mental health evolves, CBT remains a cornerstone of evidence-based practice, providing hope and support to those dealing with the complexities of varied psychological difficulties.

CHAPTER 6
CBT FOR SPECIAL POPULATIONS

Cognitive Behavioral Therapy (CBT) is a widely utilized and empirically validated treatment method that has proven helpful in a variety of demographics. However, when applying CBT to particular populations such as children and adolescents, doctors must alter their procedures to account for the age groups' distinct developmental and cognitive characteristics. Interventions in CBT for children frequently include creative and age-appropriate strategies that promote involvement, such as play therapy and art therapy. The emphasis is on reducing complicated concepts and providing tangible examples to assist children in comprehending and expressing their thoughts and emotions.

Furthermore, taking family dynamics into account is critical when tailoring therapies for children, understanding the interdependence of familial interactions and their impact on a child's cognitive and emotional development.

CBT is tailored to the unique difficulties and changes that come with adolescence. Adolescents frequently struggle with identity formation, peer interactions, and scholastic expectations. Adolescent CBT interventions may include analyzing and addressing faulty cognitive patterns about self-esteem, body image, and social interactions. Incorporating technology, such as online platforms or mobile apps, helps improve interaction with this tech-savvy demographic. Furthermore, developing a collaborative and sympathetic therapy connection is critical for providing a secure environment for teenagers to communicate their problems and strive toward meaningful change.

Moving on to older persons, CBT therapies must account for the distinctive cognitive and physical changes that come with age. Cognitive decline, memory difficulties, and concomitant medical illnesses may limit the effectiveness of typical CBT treatments. Modifications may include reducing language, using memory aids, and incorporating mindfulness and relaxation techniques. Furthermore, addressing themes of loss, sorrow, and adjusting to life transitions is critical in the context of CBT for older individuals. The therapeutic approach may include addressing and reforming dysfunctional thought patterns about aging, mortality, and a sense of purpose in later life.

Couples and family therapy within the context of CBT broadens the application of cognitive-behavioral principles to interpersonal interactions. In working with couples, CBT investigates how individual cognitions influence relationship dynamics and conflicts. The goal is to recognize and change problematic thought processes and communication approaches that perpetuate unfavorable relationships. Cognitive restructuring exercises, communication skill training, and behavioral experiments may be used as interventions to test and challenge dysfunctional relationship assumptions.

Family therapy, on the other hand, broadens the scope to encompass numerous people within a family unit. CBT in family therapy emphasizes systemic patterns of communication and behavior, stressing the reciprocal influence that family members have on one another. Interventions frequently involve investigating family roles, expectations, and communication patterns that lead to relational problems. Collaborative goal-setting and problem-solving are essential components for establishing a shared understanding of the family's issues and working toward mutually acceptable solutions.

In both couples and family therapy, the therapist's responsibility is to provide a secure and nonjudgmental environment for open discussion and examination of underlying difficulties. Furthermore, understanding and validating the diversity of family structures and dynamics is critical in adapting CBT interventions to the unique needs of each family unit.

Cultural Considerations in CBT

Cultural competence is an essential component of providing effective CBT since people from different backgrounds contribute their own perspectives, values, and coping mechanisms to the therapeutic process. Recognizing the impact of culture on the expression and interpretation of thoughts and emotions is critical in developing CBT interventions that are culturally sensitive and relevant. In terms of cultural factors in CBT, therapists must be mindful of their cultural prejudices and work constantly to understand their clients' cultural contexts.

Cultural variables may influence how mental health concerns are conceptualized, how people seek treatment, and whether certain therapy approaches are acceptable. Therapists must openly discuss their clients' cultural views and experiences to build a collaborative and culturally responsive therapy alliance. Changing the language, metaphors, and examples used in CBT sessions can improve the accessibility and effectiveness of therapies for people from different cultures.

Furthermore, incorporating cultural values and traditions into the therapeutic process might increase the relevance and acceptability of CBT. Respect for diversity and a willingness to incorporate cultural viewpoints into treatment plans help to create a more inclusive and effective therapy experience. Furthermore, continued training and supervision in cultural competency are required for therapists to continuously improve their skills in interacting with clients from diverse cultural backgrounds.

Finally, CBT with specific populations requires a sophisticated and adaptive strategy that takes into account each group's particular traits and requirements. Whether working with children, adolescents, older adults, couples, families, or individuals from various cultural origins, clinicians who use CBT must adjust their interventions to their clients' developmental, relational, and cultural subtleties. This method not only improves the efficacy of CBT but also fosters a more inclusive and client-centered therapeutic experience.

CHAPTER 7
INTEGRATION WITH OTHER THERAPEUTIC APPROACHES

Cognitive Behavioral Therapy (CBT) is widely recognized and accepted as an effective technique for treating a variety of psychiatric illnesses. However, it is not commonplace for therapists to combine CBT with other therapeutic techniques to improve overall treatment outcomes. This integration enables a more thorough and individualized approach to meeting the different needs of individuals. In this context, we will look at the integration of CBT with psychopharmacology, psychodynamic therapy, Acceptance and Commitment Therapy (ACT), and holistic treatments.

Cognitive behavioral therapy and psychopharmacology

The combination of CBT and psychopharmacology is a multifaceted approach to addressing mental health issues. Psychopharmacology employs drugs to treat symptoms, whereas CBT focuses on changing dysfunctional thought patterns and behaviors. The combination of these two techniques can be especially effective for people suffering from depression, anxiety, or schizophrenia. Psychotropic drugs can alleviate acute symptoms quickly, making the setting more suitable for cognitive restructuring and behavioral interventions guided by CBT. However, maintaining a collaborative and communicative connection between the prescribing psychiatrist and the CBT therapist is critical for ensuring a cohesive treatment plan. This combination recognizes the biological basis of mental health issues while addressing cognitive and behavioral elements using CBT approaches.

<u>CBT and psychodynamic therapy:</u>

The combination of CBT and psychodynamic therapy brings together two separate but compatible therapeutic techniques. Psychodynamic therapy investigates the unconscious processes and unresolved conflicts that drive current behavior, whereas cognitive behavioral therapy focuses on recognizing and altering maladaptive thought patterns and actions. Integrating these approaches can be extremely effective when dealing with deep-seated issues that cause continuous psychological pain. Psychodynamic insights can help to understand underlying problems, whilst CBT procedures provide practical skills for addressing and changing harmful behaviors. This integration necessitates a trained therapist who can move between the depth-oriented investigation of psychodynamic therapy and the organized, goal-oriented therapies of cognitive behavioral therapy. It focuses on gaining a full understanding of the individual, integrating insight-oriented study with active transformation tactics.

<u>CBT with ACT (Acceptance and Commitment Therapy):</u>

The combination of CBT and Acceptance and Commitment Therapy (ACT) is a hybrid of cognitive and mindfulness-based techniques. CBT focuses on confronting and modifying harmful thought patterns, whereas ACT stresses accepting thoughts and emotions, fostering mindfulness, and committing to values-based behaviors. This integration acknowledges the importance of both acceptance and transformation tactics in improving psychological well-being.

By incorporating mindfulness practices, people can learn to observe and accept their thoughts and feelings without judgment, laying the groundwork for cognitive restructuring within the CBT paradigm. Furthermore, ACT's emphasis on values-based activities complements CBT's goal-oriented approach, resulting in a more comprehensive understanding of personal fulfillment and life satisfaction. This integration enables a flexible and tailored therapy approach that meets each client's specific demands.

Integrating cognitive behavioral therapy (CBT) into holistic approaches

The holistic integration of CBT entails merging cognitive and behavioral interventions within a broader framework that takes the individual as a whole—mind, body, and spirit.

This approach acknowledges the interdependence of many facets of well-being, such as physical health, lifestyle, and personal beliefs. Holistic treatments frequently combine CBT with mindfulness, meditation, yoga, and nutritional therapy.

This integration seeks to enhance total wellness and resilience by addressing the physical, emotional, and spiritual aspects of a person's life. Holistic CBT acknowledges the influence of lifestyle factors on mental health and includes tactics for improving self-care and self-awareness. The incorporation into holistic approaches emphasizes the necessity of addressing the individual as a whole, recognizing the reciprocal interaction of cognitive-behavioral processes and larger life settings.

To summarize, the integration of CBT with other therapeutic techniques indicates the changing character of psychiatric treatment. Using CBT in conjunction with psychopharmacology, psychodynamic therapy, ACT, or holistic techniques allows therapists to provide more nuanced and targeted therapies.

This integration enables a thorough awareness of each individual's specific needs, resulting in a more holistic and successful approach to mental health therapy.

Therapists should carefully evaluate each client's unique qualities and the nature of their presenting concerns when determining the best combination of therapy modalities for optimal treatment outcomes.

CHAPTER 8
ETHICAL AND PROFESSIONAL ISSUES IN CBT

Confidentiality and boundaries:

Confidentiality is fundamental to the therapeutic relationship, and Cognitive Behavioral Therapy (CBT) is no different. Therapists must respect the confidentiality of information supplied by clients during sessions, fostering an environment in which clients feel comfortable disclosing personal and sensitive information. Confidentiality is critical for developing trust and maintaining a therapeutic connection, as clients are more inclined to open up when they believe their information will be protected. However, maintaining confidentiality can be difficult, especially when legal or ethical duties oblige therapists to violate it. For example, if there is a danger of harm to the client or others, therapists may need to communicate information with appropriate persons while balancing the duty to protect against the obligation to maintain confidentiality.

Boundaries in CBT refer to the distinct separation of the professional and personal parts of the therapy relationship. Establishing and maintaining proper boundaries is critical to keeping the therapeutic environment focused on the client's well-being. Therapists should avoid dual partnerships, in which they play numerous roles with a client, which could jeopardize impartiality and professional judgment. Furthermore, therapists must be conscious of the power dynamics that exist in the therapeutic interaction and avoid using their position for personal gain. Finding a balance between empathy and professionalism is critical for creating a therapeutic atmosphere in which clients feel supported while adhering to the ethical standards of CBT.

<u>Informed consent:</u>

Informed consent is a core ethical tenet in CBT that requires clients to have a thorough grasp of the therapy process, goals, and potential risks and benefits. Therapists must offer clients detailed information regarding the nature of CBT, the strategies used, and what to expect during the therapeutic process.

This transparency enables clients to make informed decisions regarding their participation in therapy while also encouraging collaboration between the therapist and the client. Informed consent is an ongoing process, which means that therapists should keep clients informed about any changes in treatment procedures and acquire their approval before introducing new interventions.

In CBT, informed consent includes the use of technology in therapy, such as online platforms or electronic communication. Therapists must teach clients about the possible risks of using technology in treatment, including issues of privacy and confidentiality. Clients should also be told about the limitations of online therapy and given the option of choosing whether or not they are comfortable with this kind of treatment. Respecting and sustaining the idea of informed consent ensures that clients actively participate in their treatment and feel empowered in decision-making.

<u>Cultural competence:</u>

Cultural competency is an important part of ethical and professional practice in CBT, emphasizing the need for therapists to understand and respect their clients' different cultural origins. Culture influences people's views, values, and communication methods, all of which can have a substantial impact on the therapeutic process. Therapists must be mindful of their cultural prejudices and constantly educate themselves about other cultural norms to give effective and sympathetic care to clients from various backgrounds.

Cultural competency in CBT refers to the adaptation of therapy interventions to the client's cultural setting. This may entail changing vocabulary, considering cultural metaphors, and acknowledging the influence of cultural influences on emotional and behavioral expression. Additionally, therapists should be aware of the role of cultural stigma about mental health and collaborate with clients to address any cultural obstacles that may impede the therapeutic process. Integrating cultural competency into CBT ensures that therapy is relevant, respectful, and tailored to each client's specific requirements, resulting in a more inclusive and effective therapeutic setting.

<u>Continued Education and Supervision:</u>

Continuous learning and supervision are essential components of CBT's ethical and professional practices. Therapists are encouraged to participate in ongoing education to stay current on the newest developments in the area, such as new research findings, developing treatment practices, and advances in understanding mental health.

This dedication to continuous education ensures that therapists serve their clients with the most up-to-date and evidence-based interventions possible, hence improving service quality.

Supervision is another important part of professional development in CBT. Regular supervision sessions provide an opportunity for therapists to discuss situations, seek help, and receive critical feedback from more experienced professionals. This collaborative process encourages therapists to reflect on their practice, identify areas for development, and improve their professional skills. Furthermore, supervision protects against therapist fatigue by providing emotional support and limiting the accumulation of unresolved issues in the therapy process.

<u>Self-care for therapists:</u>

CBT emphasizes the importance of self-care, understanding that therapists must maintain their well-being to provide effective and ethical care to clients. Therapists frequently face emotional and psychological problems in their work, such as dealing with client trauma, maintaining therapeutic boundaries, and dealing with the intensity of emotional disclosures. Prioritizing self-care practices can help therapists avoid burnout, compassion fatigue, and emotional tiredness.

Therapists' self-care consists of several facets, including physical, emotional, social, and spiritual health.

Regular physical activity, keeping a healthy work-life balance, and seeking assistance from coworkers are all important aspects of self-care. Therapists must also develop self-awareness and mindfulness to regulate the emotional impact of their profession and avoid the accumulation of vicarious trauma. Establishing clear boundaries between professional and home life, taking frequent breaks, and seeking supervision when necessary are all practical measures that help therapists maintain their general well-being.

CONCLUSION

The ethical and professional issues in Cognitive Behavioral Therapy (CBT) are critical to the therapy process's effectiveness and integrity. Confidentiality and boundaries create a safe setting in which clients can share their experiences, whereas informed consent encourages collaborative decision-making. Cultural competency promotes tolerance and sensitivity to other origins, resulting in more targeted and effective responses. Continuing education and supervision are required for therapists to keep current and reflect on their profession, while self-care protects against burnout and ensures that therapists deliver the best possible care. Upholding these principles in CBT not only fulfills the profession's ethical standards, but also strengthens the therapeutic partnership, resulting in better outcomes for clients.